EAT YOURSELF THIN

David Holmer

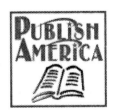

PublishAmerica
Baltimore

Hardcover 978-1-4512-9131-5
Softcover 978-1-4489-4023-3
PUBLISHED BY PUBLISHAMERICA, LLLP
www.publishamerica.com
Baltimore

Printed in the United States of America

FOREWORD

First of all, I am no doctor or nutritionist. My only education is the nutritional chapter back in 7th grade science class and what I learned in a college biology course. I do have over 40 years of life experience, struggling with weight issues. I was underweight a third of my life. Then, my weight yoyo—ed from thin to husky back and forth. Over the past decade, my weight has increased from slightly overweight to over 250 pounds with a waist of 50 inches!

I was embarrassed. None of my clothes fit me. I found myself wearing the same pajama pants, stretched out to the max, every day. I looked in the mirror one day and said, "I've had enough!" I started a daily journal of exactly what I ate and what I did. My life consisted of sleeping, watching television, internet and eating. Now, most of my inactivity is due to a disability; and, this is something that I can not change. So, I needed to focus on things that I could change.

At first, I felt overwhelmed by what I was asking of myself. I had trouble focusing. I turned off the television and computer. Suddenly, I got up and started pacing, trying to work out a solution in my mind. It dawned on me... I was exercising! It wasn't much, but it was what I could do. I would simply pace back and forth when I could and rest when I couldn't. With exercise addressed, I had an even bigger obstacle before me: my love of food.

I took a good long look at what I was eating and asked myself, "Why?" I would load up on snack foods in the middle of the day, because I usually skipped breakfast. A little bit later, I would eat a couple sandwiches with meat and cheese because I was hungry for real food. I ate enough for two people at dinner because I craved to have that full feeling. At night, I had to have something sweet, because it seems to be the only thing that comforts me or makes me feel good. Most of all, I crave fast foods because it's quick, cheap and tastes good.

Again, it dawned on me. All the previous diets, that I have ever tried before, failed because they tried to change how I eat. How I eat is Who I am. You can NOT change who you are! But, you CAN change what you eat. Suddenly, I was no longer missing television or the internet. I was too busy finding ways to change what I was eating. I thought, I would love it if vegetables tasted just as good as fast food. Then, I decided to take on the fast food cravings!

These simple changes has helped me to lose more than 30 pounds and 7" off of my waist. I have found a couple more creative ways to exercise. I side—step back and forth in my pacing. I also like to put on music and add kicks and turns for a dancier version of pacing. I have only watched television once in the past two months—for the Superbowl game. My internet use is now down to correspondence only. And, I look in the mirror and can smile at myself.

BEVERAGES

I grew up, running out the door and barely catching the school bus. I didn't mind skipping breakfast. It was worth it, especially if I got an extra 5—10 minutes longer sleeping in! By the time I started going to highschool, I was up very early, getting ready. I still skipped breakfast. The thought of eating something, when you first get up, didn't settle well with me. It still doesn't.

The first problem I have with diets is that they try to get you to eat a breakfast. As if I don't have a calorie problem to deal with already, let's just tack on a few hundred against me to start the day! This just plainly doesn't make any sense. But, I do have to have my coffee. I love my coffee and my flavored creamers. But, I was blown away when I realized that my coffee calories were the same as one of those diet breakfasts!

I made a change. I bought flavored coffees that represented the different creamers that I liked. I started drinking the coffees black. I was amazed because, within a week, I didn't miss my creamers. I had cut almost 300 calories from my diet without missing a thing! The only drawback was that I couldn't adjust the amount of cinnamon or vanilla I wanted. I started making my own teas.

Vanilla Tea

1 Vanilla Bean

Place the bean in a pot with 1 gallon of water.
Bring to a boil. Simmer 2 hours. Serve warm.

Cinnamon Tea

2 Cinnamon Sticks

Place the sticks in a pot with 1 gallon of water.
Bring to a boil. Simmer 2 hours. Serve warm.

Clove Tea

6—8 Whole Cloves

Place the cloves in a pot with 1 gallon of water.
Bring to a boil. Simmer an hour. Serve warm.

Ginger Tea

1" Ginger Root, minced

Place the ginger in a pot with 1 gallon of water.
Bring to a boil. Simmer an hour. Serve warm.

Tea of Beet Greens

1 bunch Beet Greens, fresh

Wash and de—stem greens. Chop into 1/2" pieces.
Place the greens in a pot with 1 gallon of water.
Bring to a boil. Simmer 15 minutes. Strain and
serve.

Mint Tea

1 bunch Mint Leaves, fresh

Place the mint in a pot with 1 gallon of water.
Bring to a boil. Simmer 15 minutes. Serve warm.

Lime Tea

1 tsp Lime Zest

Run water through coffee pot or heat on stove.
Place zest in cup. Fill with water. Steep 5 minutes.

SNACKS

I grew up on snacks. In fourth grade, I would load my lunchbox up with anything snack—like that I could find. If we didn't have it, I would improvise, even if it meant using something healthy. I wanted quantity and variety. I would go so far as to hard—boil a couple of eggs, pop some popcorn, make some carrot sticks and fill some celery with peanut butter. I loved my snacks. I still do.

One problem I have with diets is that they either try to eliminate snacks or limit them to just a teaser. Whenever I tried to eliminate snacks, I would do good for a few days. But then, I would get these insatiable cravings that would end up with me blowing my diet. I never could limit myself, either. I'm sorry; but, once I start, I have trouble stopping! But, I was troubled when I realized how much calories and saturated fat I was taking in with my snacking.

I made another change. I focused on what I loved about a snack and took out what I didn't like nutritionally. I started eating my salsas and dips with vegetables. I was amazed because I didn't miss the crackers or chips. The only drawback was that raw vegtables were hard and lacked that cooked salty taste from being baked or deep—fried. I started cooking the vegetables.

Bell Pepper "Chips"

2 Bell Peppers

Halve and core peppers. Quarter each half into "chips".

Start a pot of water to boil. Fill second pot with ice and water.

Put chips into boiling water for 20 seconds. Lift out with seive.

Drop into ice water. Pull off loose skin. Dry on paper towel.

Quick Salsa

1 Tomato, diced
1 Onion, chopped
1 Jalapeno, diced
1 clove Garlic, chopped
1 tsp Lime Juice
Cilantro, minced

Mix ingredients together. Serve with Bell Pepper Chips.

Zucchini "Crackers"

1 Zucchini, peeled

Cut zucchini crosswise to form circular "crackers".
Arrange single layer on plate. Microwave for 20
seconds. Cool.

Tofu—Onion Dip

1 pkg Tofu, lowest calorie available
1 pkg Onion Soup Mix

In food processor or blender, Mix well.
Serve with Zucchini Crackers.

Jalapeno Poppers

12 Jalapeno Peppers
Tofu—Onion Dip

Halve and seed peppers. Fill with Tofu—Onion
Dip.
Place on cookie sheet. Bake for 1 hour at 325.

Onion Rings

1 large Onion
1 T Olive Oil

Cut onion into rings. Pour oil on onions. Toss to coat.

Place on cookie sheet. Bake for 45 minutes at 325.

Mushrooms

1 box Mushrooms
1 T Olive Oil

Wipe off mushrooms. Pour oil on them. Toss to coat.

Place on cookie sheet. Bake for 30 minutes at 350.

Eggplant Seasoned Fries

1 Eggplant
1 T Olive Oil
Seasoned Salt

Peel and cut eggplant into "fries". Pour oil on them. Toss to coat. Layer on cookie sheet. Sprinkle with salt.

Bake for 20 minutes at 425.

Green Bean Sticks

1 qt Green Beans
1 T Olive Oil
Sea Salt

Wash and snap beans. Pour oil on them. Toss to coat.

Place on cookie sheet. Salt. Bake for 15 at 425.

SOUPS

I grew up actually enjoying vegetables with loads of butter. I learned to cook at an early age, and my favorite recipe was from a Walt Disney cookbook. Essentially, it was lots of carrots with lots of butter with lots of brown sugar. And, that is how I loved my vegetables with lots of butter and lots of something else to make it "pop". I still do.

The problem I have with diets is that they stress the importance of vegetables but then take away the butter. I tried to eat vegetables without all the butter. It just doesn't do it for me. I would rather just skip the vegetables and save the calories. And, these butter sprays don't work either. It is more than just the taste. I like my vegetables swimming in butter. But, they do have one point—butter and margarines are full of calories and unwanted fats.

I made another change. I bought every vegetable that I was unfamiliar with. I started eating these vegetables with no butter or added seasonings. I was amazed because I found quite a few that I enjoyed without butter, particularly greens. They seemed to range from mild to very peppery in tastes without any additional seasonings. The only drawback was that I couldn't quite replace the idea of melted butter, until I flavored the cooking water. I started making my own soups.

Cream of Celery

2 c Water
2 tsp Chicken Boullion
1/2 tsp Garlic, crushed
1 tsp Celery Seeds
2 c Celery, chopped
1/4 c Skim Milk

Bring water, boullion, garlic and seeds to a boil.
Add celery. Cover and return to a boil.
Turn off heat. Let simmer on burner 15 minutes.
Remove from burner. Stir in milk. Serve warm.

Spicy Spinach Soup

2 c Water
2 tsp Beef Boullion
1/2 tsp Garlic, crushed
1/8 tsp Red Pepper Flakes
2 c Chopped Spinach, frozen

Bring water, boullion, garlic and flakes to a boil.
Add Spinach. Cover and return to a boil.
Remove from heat. Let rest 5 minutes. Serve warm.

Cream of Cucumber

2 c Water
2 tsp Chicken Boullion
1/2 tsp Garlic, crushed
1 tsp Chives
1 tsp Parsley Flakes
2 c Cucumbers, peeled and diced
1/4 c Skim Milk

Bring water, boullion, garlic and herbs to a boil.
Add cucumbers. Cover and return to a boil.
Turn off heat. Let simmer on burner 15 minutes.
Remove from burner. Stir in milk. Serve warm.

Mustard Greens Soup

2 c Water
2 tsp Beef Boullion
1/2 tsp Garlic, crushed
2 c Chopped Mustard Greens, frozen
1/8 tsp Nutmeg
1/4 c Skim Milk

Bring water, boullion and garlic to a boil.
Add greens and nutmeg. Cover and return to a boil.
Remove from heat. Let rest. Stir in milk. Serve.

Swiss Chard Soup

2 c Water
2 tsp Chicken Boullion
1/2 tsp Garlic, crushed
1/2 tsp Minced Onion
2 c Swiss Chard Leaves, chopped
1 T Lemon Juice

Bring water, boullion, garlic and onion to a boil.
Add chard. Cover and return to a boil.
Turn off heat. Let simmer on burner for 15 minutes.
Remove from burner. Stir in juice. Serve warm.

Bok Choy Soup

1 large Bok Choy
2 c Water
2 tsp Beef Boullion
1/2 tsp Garlic, crushed
1 tsp Sesame Seeds

Wash and de-stem bok choy. Cut stem in 1 " pieces.
In fry pan, toast sesame seeds. Chop bok choy leaves.
Bring water, boullion, garlic and stems to a boil.
Simmer for 10 minutes. Add leaves. Cover and turn off heat.
Remove from burner. Stir in sesame. Serve warm.

Zucchini and Mint

2 c Water
2 tsp Chicken Boullion
1 T Mint, minced
2 c Zucchini, diced

Bring water, boullion and mint to a boil.
Add zucchini. Cover and return to a boil.
Turn off heat. Let simmer on burner 15 minutes.
Serve warm.

Mushrooms and Bok Choy

2 c Water
2 tsp Beef Boullion
1/2 tsp Garlic, crushed
1 c Mushrooms, sliced
1 c Bok Choy, chopped

Bring water, boullion and garlic to a boil.
Add mushrooms and bok choy. Cover.
Simmer 15 minutes. Serve warm.

SALADS

I grew up with a mom who didn't much care for lettuce. For us, a salad was a bunch of raw vegetables drenched in a delicious salad dressing. My favorite salad of all time is my aunt's broccoli and cauliflower covered with a sugary mayonnaise dressing. Like I said before, I don't mind vegetables and loved it when they were drenched. And, of course, I still do.

I finally have some common ground with diets. I have no problem cutting out those "extras" most people like to put on top of a plate of lettuce, like ham and cheeses. If you don't like the taste of lettuce, don't start with it on your plate. I also have no problem using all those low calorie salad dressings to pour on my vegetables. However, these diets assume that you will use only a tablespoon of dressing. The amounts that I use bring that salad right back up in calories.

I needed to make another change. Manufacturing companies have already done a fantastic job of taking my favorite dressings from 130 calories to 60 calories per serving. I needed to get creative and bring these dressings all the way down to the lowest calories possible. I started making my own dressings. From these dressings, I created great salad combinations.

Garlic Pepper Cream

Black Peppercorns
1/4 c Onion
1 T Garlic, crushed
1/4 c Skim Milk

Freshly grind out 1/8 tsp of pepper. Place in processor.
Add remaining ingredients. Mix until completely blended.

Cucumber Salad

1 Cucumber
Garlic Pepper Cream

Peel and dice cucumber. Drench in cream. Serve.
(for a spicy alternative, add a dash of cayenne)

Zucchini and Mushrooms

1 c Zucchini, chopped
1 c Mushrooms, chopped
Garlic Pepper Cream

Mix vegetables. Drench in cream. Serve.
(for an alternative, microwave veggies for warm salad)

Chicken Vinaigrette

1 c Water
1 tsp Chicken Boullion
1/2 tsp Garlic, crushed
1/4 c Onion
1/4 c Vinegar
1 T Olive Oil

Heat water and boullion just enough to dissolve. Cool.
In food processor, mix ingredients completely.

Bell Pepper Salad

1 Green Bell Pepper, diced
1 Red Bell Pepper, diced
1 Yellow Bell Pepper, diced
Chicken Vinaigrette

Mix vegetables. Drench in vinaigrette. Serve.
(for a spicy alternative, add a diced jalapeno)

Swiss Chard and Red Onion

1 bunch Swiss Chard, chopped
1 large Red Onion, chopped
Chicken Vinaigrette

Mix vegetables. Drench in vinaigrette. Serve.

Sweet Mustard Sauce

1/2 c Mustard
1 c Water
1 pkt Saccharin

In shaker, blend ingredients together. Shake well.

Celery Salad

2 c Celery, chopped
1 tsp Dill Weed
Sweet Mustard Sauce

Mix celery and dill. Drench in sauce. Serve.

Spinach Citrus Salad

2 c Spinach, chopped
1 tsp lemon zest
1 tsp lime zest
Sweet Mustard Sauce

Mix spinach and zests. Drench in sauce. Serve.

Beef Vinaigrette

1 c Water
1 tsp Beef Boullion
1/2 tsp Ginger, crushed
1/4 c Onion
1/4 c Vinegar
1 T Olive Oil

Heat water and boullion just enough to dissolve. Cool.
In food processor, mix ingredients completely.

Bok Choy Salad

2 c Bok Choy, chopped
1/8 tsp Garlic, crushed
Beef Vinaigrette

Mix bok choy and garlic. Drench in vinaigrette. Serve.

Mustard Greens with Jalapenos

2 c Mustard Greens, chopped
1 Jalapeno, diced
Beef Vinaigrette

Mix greens and jalapeno. Drench in vinaigrette. Serve.

SIDES

I grew up on large family dinners of meat, potatoes and corn or spaghetti with meatballs and garlic bread. Our family was also a huge fan of casseroles. Our vegetables were primarily potatoes and corn, considered more as starches today. The closest thing to a vegetable side would be green bean casserole at Thanksgiving, another great big meal. I loved large dinners. I still do.

My fourth problem with diets are these extremely small portions. If I didn't have my large dinner, I would be irritable and unsatisfied. Another thing I don't understand about diets: Ever since 7th grade, we are taught about the food chart. Remember, 1—2—3—4—5—6, fats—dairy—meat—fruit—vegetable—cereal? Well, where is it in all these diets. Most of the servings have disappeared. They also seem to be off balance from what we teach our children. Now, I agree that serving sizes are smaller portions than what we might think, so…

I made some changes. I had to. When I looked at the actual serving sizes that I was eating in this large meal, I found 6 meat servings and 12 cereal servings. This is double of what I need for the whole day. I needed to cut these amounts in half. Each typical plate was 1/2 meat and 1/2 cereal, bread or other starch. I decided to cut my meat portion to 1/4, cut my cereal portion to 1/4, and fill the other half of each plate with some low calorie vegetables. I started making my own vegetable sides.

Roasted Celery Hearts

2 Celery Hearts
Olive Oil

Rub oil on celery. Place on cookie sheet.
Bake in oven for 1 hour at 350. Serve warm.

Asian Spinach Sautee

1 T Peanut Oil
1" piece Ginger Root, minced
4 c Spinach, chopped
1 T Sesame Seeds, toasted

Heat oil in sauce pan. Sautee ginger for 3 minutes.
Add spinach and sesame. Sautee 3 minutes. Serve.

Spicy Pickled Cucumbers

1 T Olive Oil
1 tsp Red Pepper Flakes
1/2 tsp Garlic, crushed
4 Cucumbers, peeled and sliced
1 T Lime Juice

Heat oil in sauce pan. Sautee flakes for 2 minutes.
Add garlic. Sautee for 2 minutes. Add cucumbers.
Sautee for 1 minute. Let cool. Place in container.
Add juice. Stir. Cover. Refrigerate. Serve cold.

Mustard Greens Chili

1 T Olive Oil
1 tsp Red Pepper Flakes
1 tsp Cumin Seeds
4 c Mustard Greens, chopped
1 tsp Ground Cumin
1 tsp Chili Powder

Heat oil in sauce pan. Sautee flakes and seeds for 2 minutes.
Add greens and spices. Sautee 3 minutes.
Serve with Garlicky Tomato Sauce.

Garlicky Tomato Sauce

1 Tomato, chopped
1 T Garlic, crushed
1 pkt Saccharin

In food processor, blend ingredients together. Mix well.

Stuffed Green Peppers

4 Green Bell Peppers
1 c Celery, chopped
1 c Onion, chopped
1 c Zucchini, chopped
1 c Mushrooms, chopped
1 T Italian Seasoning
Garlicky Tomato Sauce

Wash and cut off tops of peppers. Carefully seed peppers.

Set peppers on cookie sheet. If they roll, trim bottoms of pepper.

In bowl mix vegetables and seasoning. Stuff peppers equally.

Spoon sauce over tops to cover. Bake for 1 hour at 350. Serve.

Swiss Chard with Citrus

1 T Olive Oil
4 c Swiss Chard, chopped
1 T Lime Zest
1 T Lemon Zest
1 T Lime Juice

Heat oil in sauce pan. Sautee chard stems for 5 minutes.

Add zests. Sautee for 1 minute. Add chard leaves. Sautee for 3 minutes. Remove from heat. Add juice. Serve warm.

DESSERTS

One of the funniest memories I have is growing up cooking desserts. I decided to make oatmeal cookies one night for our family. I was following the recipe on the back of the oatmeal can. Somehow, I got distracted and started following the recipe below it. When the first batch of cookies came out, my dad asked, "What are these green things?" I said, "Green Peppers." My cookies had finely chopped onions and green peppers in them. I started following the recipe for a meatloaf! I was quite young at the time and didn't realize the mistake.

Besides cooking, I grew up enjoying baking. There's is nothing better at the end of the day than going into the kitchen and baking some fantastic dessert. Sure, I have enjoyed the occasional scoop of ice cream late at night. But, it does not compare to having fresh baked chocolate cake from scratch or a warm slice of apple pie. I loved my baked desserts. I still do.

Once again, diets disappoint me with their version of a dessert. Usually, they just give you an apple or tell you to eat a serving of fruit. Sometimes, you are out of luck because they already gave that serving to you for breakfast, lunch or as a snack. The reasoning behind cutting out the baked goods is the huge calorie count in flour, sugars, butters and creams. The drawback to eating just a serving of fruit is that it lacks the baked good tastes and feelings from eating something warm and delicious. So, I started making my own desserts.

Blueberries and "Cream"

1 pt Blueberries
1 tsp Vanilla Extract

Mix berries and vanilla in microwave—safe bowl.
Microwave for 2 minutes. Stir. Serve warm.

"Candied" Pears

1 can Pear Halves, in lite syrup
1/2 tsp Ginger

Place pears and juice in microwave—safe bowl.
Sprinkle with ginger. Microwave 2 minutes. Serve.

Peach "Cobbler"

1 can Sliced Peaches, in lite syrup
1/2 tsp Cinnamon

Place peaches and juice in microwave—safe bowl.
Sprinkle with cinnamon. Microwave 2 minutes.
Serve.

"Poached" Pears

1 can Pear Halves, in lite syrup
1/2 tsp Ground Cloves

Place pears and juice in microwave—safe bowl.
Sprinkle with cloves. Microwave 2 minutes. Serve.

Sliced Apple "Pie"

1 large Red Delicious Apple
1 large Golden Delicious Apple
1 tsp Cinnamon
1 pkt Saccharin

Place apples in microwave—safe bowl. Add spices.
Toss. Microwave 6 minutes. Let cool. Serve warm.

Strawberry—Mint Soup

1 pt Strawberries, sliced
1 T Mint, minced
1 pkt Saccharin

In food processor, blend ingredients until form puree.
Place in microwave—safe bowl. Microwave 2 minutes. Serve.

CRAVINGS

I grew up on fast food. Even with all these wonderful changes, I still get my cravings about twice a week, almost every third day, for fast food. I'm talking about a whole BK meal, KFC or the 10 pack soft tacos at Taco Bell. And, if it's not for fast food, I would be craving the buffet, either Chinese or Indian. I loved going out for those quick, cheap and great tasting meals. But, guess what?! I have found a better alternative!

Diets really get it wrong when they say, "You can eat out" just change what you are eating! Like we would go out of our way to have a salad somewhere, when we can have that at home. Hello !!! Why do we go out to eat? Because of the foods we like! I have found wonderful alternatives for my five strongest cravings. I have found the answer to where all diets have failed me. I started making my own fast food cravings.

Top of the list for my favorite cravings is the Chinese Buffet. Now, I am not one of those who comes into the China Buffet and eat the saphetti, pizza and fried chicken. I come for the Chinese food! My favorite would be the egg rolls. Sometimes, I could eat a few platefuls of them, followed by a few platefuls of Stir-fry on mounds of rice. Calories and saturated fats go out the window. I want that flavor!

"Egg Roll" with Hot Mustard Sauce

1 T Olive Oil
1 pt Alfalfa Sprouts
1 c Cabbage, grated
1 T Mustard
Cayenne Pepper

Heat oil in sauce pan. Stir-fry vegetables. Plate.
Add mustard to teeny pinch of cayenne. Mix well.
Serve mustard on side of plate with veggies.
(for alternative, serve veggies with ginger root and
soy sauce)

Chinese "Beef" Stir Fry

1 c Water
2 tsp Beef Boullion
1 T Olive Oil
2 c Bok Choy
1 pt Snow Peas
Soy Sauce

Bring water and boullion to a boil. Let reduce down
to syrup.
Heat oil in sauce pan. Stir-fry vegetables for 3—5
minutes.
Remove from heat. Stir in reduced boullion. Serve
with sauce.

An extremely close second on that list of cravings is a trip to Burger King. I am a true fan of the Whopper. I want the Whopper meal, fries and vanilla milkshake included. There is just something about the way the ketchup and mayonnaise and the juicy burger just mixes into this tasty wet mess. And, I love it !!! Top it all of with fries loaded down with lots of salt. Once again, the calories and saturated fat goes out the window. I want that flavorful experience!

Quick Mayonnaise

1 Egg
Skim Milk
Dry Mustard

Hard boil egg, shell and discard yolk. Place in food processor.
Add a splash of milk and a teeny pinch of mustard. Mix into spread.

Eggplant "Hamburger" Patties

1 Eggplant, sliced 3/8" thick
Olive Oil
Salt
Pepper

Rub oil on eggplant. Salt and pepper both sides to taste.

Get grill really hot. Grill to a light brown. Turning for marks.

"Hamburger" Sandwich

2 large Portebella Mushrooms
4 T Quick Mayonnaise
1 Lettuce Leaf
1 Tomatoe Slice, 1/4" thick
1 Eggplant "Hamburger" Patty
4 T Garlicky Tomato Sauce
3 Dill Pickle Slices
1 small Onion Slice, about 6—8 rings

Remove the gills from the mushroom caps. Fill one cap with mayonnaise.

Layer with lettuce leaf and tomatoe. Fill other cap with burger.

Layer with sauce, onions and pickles. Assemble sandwich. Enjoy!

Zucchini "Fries"

1 Zucchini
1 T Olive Oil
Koshar or Sea Salt

Cut zucchini into fries. Toss with oil. Place on cookie sheet.
Sprinkle heavy with salt. Bake for 20 minutes at 425.

Skim Milk "Shake"

1 c Ice
1/3 c Dry Milk
1 c Skim Milk
1 tsp Vanilla Extract
1 pkt Saccharin

Place all ingredients in food processor. Blend into thick shake.

My second favorite buffet in the world is Indian cuisine. It is hard to find such spice in any other food to match these exquisite tastes. Calories can really add up when you consider having a dish made with coconut milk. But, there are times when I just gotta have these flavor combinations!

Indian "Spring Roll"

1 T Olive Oil
1 pt Alfalfa Sprouts
1 c Cucumber, grated
1 T Peanut Butter, chunky

Heat oil in sauce pan. Stir fry vegetables.
Stir in peanut butter until melted. Serve warm.

Indian Vegetable Curry

1 T Olive Oil
1/2 tsp Red Pepper Flakes
1/2 tsp Ginger Root, minced
1 c Celery, chopped
1/2 c Bell Pepper, chopped
1/2 c Mushrooms, chopped
2 c Zucchini, chopped
1/2 tsp cinnamon
1 T Curry Powder
1 c Skim Milk
1/2 tsp Vanilla Extract
1 pkt Saccharin

Heat oil in sauce pan. Stir fry flakes and ginger for
1 minute.
Add celery, pepper, mushrooms and zucchini. Stir Fry.
Add remaining ingredients. Mix well. Let heat
through. Serve.

My second favorite fast food in the world is KFC. I about laughed when they came out with their KFC bowls. We have been mixing our chicken, mashed potatoes, corn and gravy since I was a kid. They must have hired a retiree like my dad, who ate his meal like that. Truth be told, I am a huge favorite of their new grilled chicken. What a wonderful alternative. But, I still crave that mashed potatoes and gravy, which is what I mostly go there for nowadays.

Cauliflower Mash "Potatoes"

1 c Water
1 tsp Chicken Boullion
1 head Cauliflower, cut in florettes

Bring water and boullion to a boil. Add cauliflower. Boil 15 minutes. Let cool. Mix until thick consistency.
Serve warm with Brown Onion "Gravy".

Brown Onion "Gravy"

2 Onions, peeled
1 c Water
2 tsp Boullion
1/2 tsp Oregano
1 Bay Leaf
1/8 tsp Black Pepper

Roast Onion under broiler until blackened edges. Bring water, boullion and spices to a boil. Let reduce. Remove and discard bay leaf. Blend ingredients well.

Finally, I must admit that, about once a month, I make a run to the border. I can eat a whole 10 pack of soft tacos from Taco Bell. It's my dark little secret. Sometimes, I get carried away and order 20. I never can finish them all, but I do put in quite a good effort. The only big concern is the 10 or 20 servings of bread. Being that this is usually late night, those are on top of 12 servings from dinner! I squashed this craving with an amazing taco salad.

"Taco" Salad

1 T Olive Oil
1 tsp Cumin Seeds
1/2 tsp Garlic, crushed
2 c Onion, chopped
1 T Ground Cumin
Cayenne Pepper
Water
6 c Iceberg Lettuce, shredded

Heat oil in sauce pan. Saute seeds for 1 minute.

Add garlic and onions. Saute for 10 minutes. Stir often.

Add cumin, a teeny pinch of cayenne and a splash of water.

Stir until water evaporates. Serve on bed of lettuce.